GET
INFORMED!

GET INFORMED!

A Guidebook for Recently Diagnosed Diabetics and Their Loved Ones

SHARITA E. WARFIELD, MD

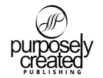

purposely created
PUBLISHING

GET INFORMED!
Published by Purposely Created Publishing Group™
Copyright © 2019 Sharita Warfield

All rights reserved.

Printed in the United States of America
ISBN: 978-1-64484-012-2

Special discounts are available on bulk quantity purchases by book clubs, associations and special interest groups. For details email: sales@publishyourgift.com or call (888) 949-6228.

For information logon to:
www.PublishYourGift.com

This book and all that I am I owe and dedicate to you, Mama.

For the unlimited advice, support, love, and encouragement you showered me with while you were here have made me who I am today, and for that I thank you.

For the unwavering strength and tenacity that you displayed as I watched you deal with adversities that life laid before you, I thank you. You pressed on gracefully as you battled diabetes and its many complications, like the warrior that you were, never once giving up or complaining, and for that I thank you. I dedicate this book to you, Gwendolyn Delores, for your greatest test in life became your testimony. It is now your testimony that I will share with the world to motivate and inspire in a positive way all while increasing the awareness of diabetes and decreasing the prevalence of its complications.

Rest well, Mama.

All my love,
Rita

Table of Contents

CHAPTER 8:

My Story

Growing up as a young girl in a single-parent home in inner city Detroit, I knew since fifth grade that I wanted to be a doctor. I had a love for science and the human body, and when my human body project won first place in the science fair it sealed the deal. My aunt and my godmother were both nurses and served as role models to me, so being in the health field was in my blood. I attended Central State University and obtained my BS in premed biology, then went to Tennessee State University and obtained my MS in microbiology. After getting my master's, I attended Wayne State University School of Medicine, where I received my MD.

While in medical school I met my husband and became pregnant with our first child during my third year. I was devastated; I thought it put a wrench in my dream of obtaining my MD for sure. Although challenging, I persevered and made it through, becoming the first doctor in my family! Yes, me, the little brown-skinned girl from Detroit! I completed my emergency medicine residency training at Howard University, then went on to complete a fellowship in medical toxicology at Wayne State University. I had two more children during my residency and fellowship. Crazy, huh? I know! It was challenging, but I can now say I worked as an EM physician for twenty-three years. During that time I served as the emergency department chairperson and medical director, along with working as an assistant clinical professor, lecturing to and training residents and fellows.

While very fulfilling, my career journey hit some low points. During my first year of residency, three months after my husband and I married, his mother passed away from gastric cancer. During my second year of residency, my mother, who was a type 2 diabetic, lost her eyesight at age fifty-seven. Her health continued to deteriorate over the years and she ultimately lost both her legs and developed kidney failure, requiring dialysis. I felt helpless, angry, and confused. How can you have a daughter that's a doctor and end up that way? I asked myself, could I have done more? I would stay on her about taking her medicine; she smoked and I would badger her to quit. I would even take her cigarettes and throw them away. I realized she wasn't eating the proper foods, so when I was home I would cook what I thought were healthy meals and make recipe suggestions to my sister, who was her primary caretaker. But ultimately, my mom died in August of 2008, three days after her birthday and two days before mine, after eleven years of battling the complications of diabetes. I was hurt that she was gone, but relieved that she wasn't suffering anymore.

Looking back on it as a physician, I realized the damage had already been done. I realized that it was my mom's responsibility to have taken better care of herself. I realized that maybe she thought she *was* taking care of herself . . . the best that she knew how. I realized that she, like so many of my African American patients with diabetes, just didn't know. They don't know the proper lifestyle changes to make. They don't know the proper foods to eat. They don't know that taking their medicine is an important part of improving their health. Maybe no one has told them what could happen or how they could end up if they don't treat their diabetes properly. Oh, sure, they've seen family members suffer, but perhaps they feel it won't happen to them.

I have also noticed that many people are unhappy with their weight. They have tried various diets and lose-weight-quick schemes and are fed up. They are frustrated that they can't reach their health goals. They may be stressed out with the demands of life and want to make a change, but don't know how. They become frustrated trying to live a healthy life.

Let me say that I truly understand and empathize. I, too, am a type 2 diabetic. After my mother passed in 2008, I was determined not to get diabetes. I got a trainer, changed my eating habits, and lost twenty-one pounds. I felt I was on my way to living my best life! But in 2010 my doctor told me I had diabetes. After having gestational diabetes in 2005 with my last child, it had come back. I was in shock! Who, me? But

I eat right, I exercise, I've lost weight, I don't "look" like a type 2 diabetic. I, too, was in denial; I refused to take the medicine at first, I said I'd just lose more weight, I'd make more dietary changes, I'd drink more water, etc. It didn't work—my hemoglobin A1c was still elevated on my next visit. I realized I had to do better. I had to practice what I preached. I had to be the change that I wanted to see. I had to do the right things to ensure that I remained healthy, so I could be around for my husband and four kids.

There is a known correlation between the food we eat and our weight gain and the development of type 2 diabetes. This is where my passion for cooking and healthy eating comes into play. As a type 2 diabetic, I had to learn the right foods to eat and the effect they had on my body. As I continue on this journey, I am still learning. I am constantly taking recipes and creatively making them into something that is healthy and tastes good. I decided to write this book to share with you my tips on how I live with diabetes and to educate those who are struggling with diabetes and weight management. I hope to impact the world in a major way.

My desire is to help as many people living with diabetes as I can. I want you to be "in the know" so you or your family members don't suffer the same fate my mother did. I want to educate you on the how, the what, and the why, so that you can improve the quality of your life and that of your family members, too. Hopefully, through my book and my 7-Step

Diabetes Management Plan, you will get the information you need to achieve the health and weight goals that you desire. You will achieve weight loss, you will require less medication, and you will be happier and ultimately have an improved quality of life. So let's join together on this health journey. My mother's story serves as my motivation; what's yours?

Introduction

As an emergency physician, it has been my life's journey to help people live and feel better. Throughout my career I have had the opportunity to see people at their best and their worst moments in life. Every day that I worked with my patients, I did my best and gave them my all to enhance their life in whatever way that I could. I treated them with dignity and respect, as I would a member of my own family. As a physician, reflecting back on the diabetic journey that my mother lived—and the many encounters I have had with similar patients—made me realize that there was a need. There was a need for further education for patients, family members, and caretakers. There was a need beyond the exam room once the diagnosis was given. There seems to be an overall disconnect, especially in certain ethnic groups like African Americans and Hispanic Americans, about the importance of treating diabetes. It is these two groups that have the highest incidence of diabetes when compared to white American adults. I felt there needed to be more dialogue, more follow-up, more accountability when it comes to managing their diabetes. I felt it was important to let them know in a way that they would understand that diabetes is a serious illness. Like hypertension, diabetes is "the other" silent killer.

There are approximately thirty million people in the United States who have diabetes, and seven million of them don't even know they have it. It is predicted that these numbers will continue to rise for years to come unless something is done. This is where my passion and purpose for writing this book comes into play. I too am a type 2 diabetic, and I was one of the seven million who didn't know I was. I decided to write this book to give you the knowledge you need and to serve as a guide on what to do now that you have been diagnosed with diabetes. I'm sharing with you many of the things that I use myself as I continue to learn to live with diabetes.

In today's world, the prevalence of weight gain, obesity, and diabetes continues to increase at an alarming rate. In most cases, the development of type 2 diabetes is related to excessive weight or weight gain. Obesity has now been declared a chronic disease. It has gripped our society in such a way that it is now an epidemic. It is even affecting our children, to the point where they have become obese and are manifesting diseases that are normally seen later in life. The reasons for the increase of society's waistline are probably multiple; however, for the most part it can be related to our food choices and to inactivity. Eating supersized portions of fast food, sodas, coffee drinks, cakes, and pies definitely contributes to the problem. Our sedentary lifestyle also contributes to the obesity problem. Technological advances have made life so convenient that they have taken the movement aspect out of things that would normally require motion to make happen.

We have electrical bicycles, self-propelling lawnmowers, robot vacuum cleaners, self-cleaning ovens, cars that drive for us, etc. You get the picture. Our children have become sedentary as well, with many opting out of outdoor games and activities to stay indoors and play computer or video games. So now is the time to do our part to put an end to this epidemic.

All is not lost; there is hope. By making the proper changes to your lifestyle and eating habits, you and your family members can be well on your way to reversing weight gain and diabetes!

In this book, *Get Informed! A Guidebook for Recently Diagnosed Diabetics and Their Loved Ones*, you will learn about the different types of diabetes, how it develops, and the complications that result when diabetes is treated poorly. You will also learn seven steps that I use to manage my diabetes that can help you and your loved ones. These steps will help you change the way you look at living with diabetes. You will receive information on various herbs and supplements that have been shown to have an additive effect when treating diabetes. You will get information on foods that will help you meet your health and weight management goals. I will also give you certain food swaps, a lot of which I use when creating my delicious, healthy meals, and so much more. It is my hope that the information contained in this book will truly change your life and the lives of your loved ones for the better.

Now is the time to take action! It is time to make a decision to live your life for the better. Make the necessary lifestyle and dietary changes that will improve your health. Make the changes that will help you combat and reverse type 2 diabetes. Make the changes that will help you lose the weight that you want to lose, reduce your hemoglobin A1c, and get your sexy back! Make the changes that will get you energized, focused, and stress free. It is my prayer that you make the changes that will allow you to "Live Your Best Life" with diabetes. I hope that the guidelines and suggestions in this book will help you to honor your body as the temple that God intended it to be. Come and join me as we embark upon this health journey together.

Sharita E. Warfield, MD

CHAPTER 1

What Is Diabetes?

Diabetes Mellitus is a chronic disease that has no cure. It is caused by the body not being able to utilize glucose the way it was intended. Scientifically, it is a result of either the beta cells in the pancreas not making enough insulin, or the body developing insulin resistance and not being able to utilize insulin as it should. "Mellitus" is Latin for "sweet." Apparently, early on the Romans would taste the urine of a patient to see if it was sweet to aid in diagnosing this condition. Thank goodness for advancements in science and the advent of tests that make that unnecessary! "Diabetes" is the Greek word for "siphon." Physicians found that patients with this condition of sweet urine would rapidly excrete ingested fluids in their urine. In other words, fluid ran through them quickly, like a siphon.

There are several types of diabetes: prediabetes, type 1 diabetes, type 2 diabetes, and gestational diabetes.

PREDIABETES

Approximately eighty-four million Americans have prediabetes; that's 1 in 3 adults, many of whom don't even know it. **Prediabetes** is when your blood sugar levels are higher than normal, but not high enough to be considered diabetic. Prediabetes develops when the body starts to have trouble utilizing insulin. **Insulin** is the hormone in the body that takes the glucose from the blood stream and allows it into cells, where it is utilized for energy. When the body doesn't use insulin correctly, this is called **insulin resistance**, which is known to be the cause of type 2 diabetes. When you go to your doctor, they will perform an **FBG**, a fasting blood glucose test, as a part of your routine checkup. This is done eight hours after your last meal, ideally in the morning. If your blood sugar level measures between 100–125 mg/dL, you have prediabetes. For nondiabetics, fasting blood sugar normally ranges between 80–99 mg/dL. Prediabetes is often not associated with any symptoms if detected early. However, diabetes develops gradually over time, and this prediabetic state is considered a risk factor for the development of type 2 diabetes. This state is where action toward a healthier way of eating and living can have the greatest impact on the prevention of the development of type 2 diabetes. Losing even just five to ten pounds can often have a significant enough effect to prevent the development of type 2 diabetes.

TYPE 1 DIABETES

Type 1 diabetes is when the cells within the pancreas don't make insulin. It is caused by an autoimmune reaction, which means the body attacks itself. During this attack, the beta cells within the pancreas are damaged, thus leading to little or no insulin production. Formerly known as insulin dependent or juvenile diabetes, type 1 diabetes is mostly diagnosed in children, teens, and young adults. Diagnosis in adulthood is rare, but can occur.

Type 1 diabetics require insulin to be placed in the body daily to be able to utilize glucose for energy. This is done by injection, i.e. giving yourself a shot, or by an insulin pump, where the insulin is delivered continuously through a catheter placed under your skin. And no, the catheter is not a needle, as many of my patients think. It is the plastic piece left behind after the needle is removed. Insulin can't be taken in a pill form because the stomach acid would break it down before it reached the bloodstream. Consult with your doctor to see which method is right for you.

The symptoms associated with Type 1 Diabetes are:

▶ Frequent urination

▶ Increase in thirst

▶ Unexplained weight loss

- Increase in appetite

- Numbness in hands or feet

- Blurry vision

- Feeling tired

- Wounds that heal slowly

- Nausea, vomiting, and abdominal pain

Unlike type 2 diabetes, patients with type 1 diabetes can develop symptoms within a few weeks to a few months after the damage to the pancreas occurs. Most of the patients that I have diagnosed with type 1 diabetes presented with severe nausea, vomiting, and abdominal pain, and are often very dehydrated. Unfortunately, there is no cure for type 1 diabetes and it can't be reversed; however, you can live a long and productive life. As most type 1 patients are children or young adults, it can be challenging when they're faced with all the food choices that their friends and peers normally eat. It will take the support of their parents, family, and friends to help them manage their diabetes. If you have type 1 diabetes, it is important to learn as much as you can about diabetes and managing your blood glucose levels.

TYPE 2 DIABETES

Previously known as adult onset or non-insulin dependent diabetes, type 2 diabetes is when the body makes insulin, but because of insulin resistance, the cells don't respond to it like they should. Think of insulin as the gatekeeper to the cell. Normally, it lets glucose into the cell, which is then used for energy. Insulin also signals the liver and muscles to store glucose for later use; however, when that storage area is full, it sends the excess glucose to fat cells to be stored as body fat. This process continues as long as there is excess glucose being ingested. When the cells don't respond, though, your pancreas makes more and more insulin in an attempt to help get glucose into the cells. Over time the cells stop responding and the blood glucose stays elevated. This excessive accumulation of glucose continues to trigger its storage in the fat cells and the body continues to gain more and more body fat. This is how being overweight and insulin resistance are risk factors for developing type 2 diabetes.

As mentioned earlier, diabetes affects approximately thirty million Americans, and about seven million of them don't even know they have it. That is because the disease process develops gradually over years and years of excessive carbohydrate intake. Type 2 diabetes is normally diagnosed in adults in their forties; however, because of our nation's obesity epidemic, more and more young adults and children are being diagnosed with type 2 diabetes as well. It is said to be genetic, and most certainly there is a gene that is passed down through the generations that leads to the development of diabetes. However, I feel that there may be certain environmental habits that may serve as triggers, which have been passed down as well. Like Grandma's sweet potato pie, macaroni and cheese, cornbread dressing, candied yams . . . you get the picture? Well, all of those great generational recipes that have been passed down, along with an increase in the eating of processed foods and a sedentary lifestyle, lead to an increase of belly fat. This **truncal** (belly fat) **obesity** puts you at greater risk of developing type 2 diabetes.

So, what are the symptoms of type 2 diabetes? They are pretty much the same as type 1, because the end result is the same: too much sugar in the bloodstream. Since the disease progression is gradual, by the time symptoms start to appear the damage has already begun. If left uncorrected, weight gain may lead to insulin resistance, which may lead to prediabetes, which ultimately leads to type 2 diabetes. This progression can take five to ten years from first being diagnosed with prediabetes. The symptoms are:

▸ Frequent urination

▸ Increase in thirst

▸ Unexplained weight loss

▸ Increase in appetite

- ▶ Numbness in hands or feet

- ▶ Blurry vision

- ▶ Feeling tired

- ▶ Wounds that heal slowly

- ▶ Increase in number of infections

If you or your loved one has any of the above symptoms, you should visit your doctor immediately to get tested. They will perform an FBG. If your level is 126 mg/dL or higher, you have diabetes. They may also perform a **hemoglobin A1c test**. This test measures your average blood sugar level over the past three months. If you have had elevated or excess sugar in your blood, it will measure high. If it is 6.5 percent or higher, you have diabetes. Again, once diagnosed, it is very important to get help from your physician and to build a support team that will help you manage your diabetes. As you read further, I will share with you some of my personal experiences and how I manage my own type 2 diabetes.

GESTATIONAL DIABETES

Gestational diabetes occasionally develops during pregnancy in women who didn't have diabetes prior to becoming pregnant. Annually, it affects approximately 2 to 10 percent of pregnant women, with a higher tendency amongst African American, Hispanic American, and American Indian ethnic groups. During pregnancy your body goes through hormone changes and weight gain. Sometimes the changes and weight gain lead to cells becoming insulin resistant, and thus gestational diabetes develops. There are generally no symptoms with gestational diabetes. Therefore, you have to be tested. The risk factors for developing gestational diabetes include:

- Being older than twenty-five

- Having high blood pressure

- Having a family history of diabetes

- Being overweight before pregnancy

- Gaining a lot of weight during pregnancy

- Having had gestational diabetes previously

- Being pregnant with multiple babies

Your ob-gyn will perform a blood test on you around twenty-four to twenty-eight weeks, based on your history and risk factors, to test for gestational diabetes. The initial test that is done is called a glucose screening exam. If this test is positive, then you will have to be tested further. The next test is called a **glucose tolerance test**. In this test, they will initially draw your blood after you fast overnight to determine your fasting blood glucose level. You will then drink a sweet glucose-containing drink and then have your blood redrawn at one, two, and three hours afterward. You are diagnosed with gestational diabetes if at one hour your level is 180 mg/dL or higher, at two hours it's 155 mg/dL or higher, and at three hours it's 140 mg/dL or higher.

Let me share my story with you about when I took the glucose tolerance test and was ultimately diagnosed with gestational diabetes. I arrived at the office and was checked in, and my blood was drawn to check my fasting blood level. I was then given the glucose drink and told to drink it and then sit and wait for the subsequent blood draws. I opened the bottle and took the first sip of this, to me, sugar times one thousand, super-sugary drink. I am generally not a sweets eater, so maybe I'm being extra in my description, but it was very sweet. Anyway, I gulped it down and then began the waiting process.

About thirty minutes into it, I started to feel warm and tingly inside. I began to sweat a little, then became dizzy and felt like the room was spinning around me. I just knew I was going to pass out as I sat there wondering, what the heck is happening? This was my fourth pregnancy and I had never had that reaction before. I felt then that something might be wrong. The symptoms eventually went away and I didn't pass out, so I finished the next two blood draws.

The following week my doctor called me with the news that my results were abnormal and that I had gestational diabetes. I was devastated, but determined to do what I needed to do for my health, as well as that of my unborn child. I was placed on insulin and met with a dietitian who gave me healthy eating tips. At the time I thought, How do you put a pregnant woman in her third trimester on a diet? This is so unfair. But like a soldier I pressed on and did what I had to do, and ultimately I delivered a healthy baby girl. The gestational diabetes went away and all was well—or so I thought. In spite of all of my efforts, though, I was diagnosed with type 2 diabetes five years later.

CHAPTER 2

What Causes Diabetes?

As previously mentioned, type 1 diabetes is believed to be genetically passed down or caused by an autoimmune reaction. The body's immune system is designed to keep you safe. It is your defense system against infection and disease. It is unique to each individual and recognizes your cells as your own. It also identifies that which is foreign, like harmful bacteria or viruses. When a harmful germ is detected, the immune system mounts an attack against that foreign invader to destroy it. However, an **autoimmune** reaction is when your body mistakenly attacks your normal cells. In type 1 diabetes this attack occurs on the cells responsible for producing insulin.

We know that prediabetes and type 2 diabetes are related to weight gain and insulin resistance. With our nation currently living through a consistently rising obesity epidemic, it makes sense that diseases related to obesity are on the rise as well. Over ninety-three million Americans were deemed overweight or obese in 2016. It is felt that this number will continue to rise in the years to come. If you are obese it puts you at risk of developing high blood pressure, diabetes, heart disease, strokes, certain cancers, arthritis, and sleep apnea. Obesity itself is now recognized as a chronic disease by the American Medical Association and other agencies. In 2008, the estimated annual medical cost of obesity in the US was $147 billion. African Americans and Hispanic Americans have a higher rate of obesity when compared to white Americans and Asian Americans.

What is the definition of obesity? It is defined as a **BMI (Body Mass Index)** that is greater than 30. The BMI was developed as a screening tool to determine if a person is overweight.

BMI < 18.5 = underweight

BMI 18.5–24.9 = normal weight

BMI 25–29.9 = overweight

BMI 30–34.9 = obese

BMI 35–39.9 = severe obesity

BMI > 40 = morbid obesity

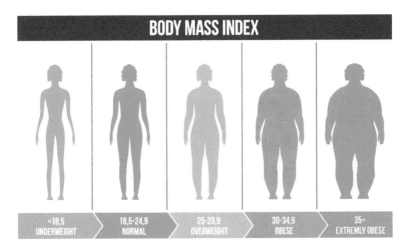

The BMI is easily calculated by multiplying your weight in pounds by 703 and dividing that by your height in inches squared.

<u>Weight (lbs.) x 703</u>
Height (in.) x Height (in.)

So let's use me as an example. I weigh 165 lbs. and I am 5'7", so what is my BMI? First, I need to convert my height into inches; there are 12 inches in a foot, so you take that and multiply it by 5, and then add the remaining inches, yielding 67 inches.

<u>165 x 703 = 115,995</u>
67x 67 = 4,489

BMI = 25.8

My BMI is 25.8, which means, according to the reference, that I am in the overweight category.

This mathematical calculation was developed over one hundred years ago to be used by health care professionals. Its usefulness has been challenged by a few modern day scientists who feel it may cause many of us to be mislabeled because of its shortcomings. The BMI doesn't differentiate between muscle and fat; as muscle weighs more than fat, a very muscular athlete would have an elevated BMI, making him or her overweight by the old standards. Also, the research that was done to derive the formula was mostly done on white men and women. Therefore it does not take into account the differing patterns of fat deposits or the muscle and bone density variations that exist in other races and ethnic groups. That being said, the BMI screening tool remains the most widely used amongst health care professionals. So until further research warrants a change, some will utilize these numbers loosely as a gauge of weight management.

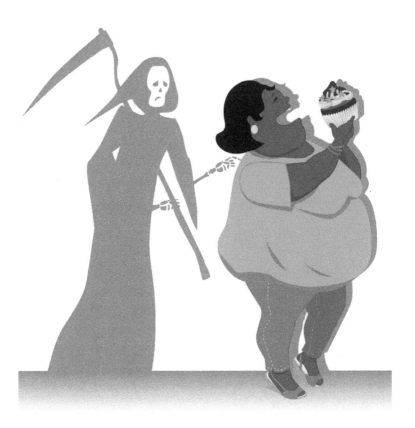

THE OBESE NATION

Why are we an obese nation? Why does weight gain and obesity continue on an upward trend? What factors lead to weight gain and obesity becoming an epidemic? Quite frankly, our society, lifestyle, and eating habits have all contributed to this widespread problem, pun intended.

Technology has made us sedentary. We spend way too much time sitting at the computer for work as well as for play. We spend countless hours in front of the TV screen, binge watching our favorite shows and eating unhealthy snacks. Many of our household chores are now done electrically or are motorized. Walking and biking as modes of transportation have been replaced with cars, and even when we drive we try and find the closest parking spot to the door. Even our children have gotten lazy and less active, many preferring to stay inside playing computer games instead of going outdoors. If it weren't for the one hour of physical education activity they get at school, many wouldn't get any exercise at all. I remember as a child growing up that I couldn't wait to go outside and would be mad when the streetlights came on. Perhaps many of you can relate? That's when Mama said you had to be home! Anyway, you get the point; we don't get enough physical activity to burn off the calories that we take in.

Speaking of calories in, we consume entirely too much sugar and carbohydrates, most of which is added during the processing or preparing of certain foods. A lot of foods contain hidden sugars, and you may not even realize the amount you are consuming. The low-fat food craze led to a lot more sugar being added to replace the fat and enhance the flavor. We have also become a very impatient society. We want everything fast; we are always in a hurry to get to the next big thing. In the interest of time, good home-cooked meals have been replaced with high calorie fast food choices and restaurant meals. Our portion sizes are outrageous. Most of the time, one portion is enough to feed two people. Everything is super-sized, and it keeps you wanting and coming back for more.

The marketing teams for these fast food chains play to your weaknesses as well. Have you ever noticed that about every third TV commercial is about food? Also, a lot of labeling and packaging for certain foods may be misleading to the uninformed. Whole wheat may not mean 100 percent whole wheat. Organic may not contain 100 percent organic ingredients. Gluten free doesn't mean sugar or fat free. Many people feel that gluten-free foods are healthier, but they are made for people who have Celiac disease and can't tolerate gluten. They often contain more carbohydrates per serving. Low fat doesn't necessarily mean better for you, as it often contains a lot of added sugar. Sugar free may not be sugar free.

Sugar is a crystalline substance that comes from the sugarcane and sugar beet plants. It is used as a sweetener and a preservative. We as Americans consume so much sugar that sugar addiction has become an epidemic, with the excessive consumption correlating with the rise of obesity and type 2 diabetes. It has been said that sugar is just as addicting, if not more so, as drugs and alcohol.

When we eat sugar, it releases a "feel-good" chemical in the brain called dopamine. This is known as a sugar high. The release of dopamine causes the pleasurable "high" that you experience, and you want to experience it again, so you eat more sugar. As you consume more and more sugar, though, your brain releases less and less dopamine. You will ultimately have to consume greater and greater amounts of sugar to experience the same "high" feeling. This is the vicious cycle that leads to sugar addiction. This is why eating or drinking sugar makes you crave more sugar.

The average American consumes about thirty to sixty teaspoons of sugar a day. If you think about it, a 12 oz. can of soda has about eight to ten teaspoons of sugar in it. If you drink a soda with each meal, that's thirty teaspoons right there, and we haven't even added in the sugars in the food! It is recommended that the average adult only consume six teaspoons of sugar a day. Sugar programs our bodies to gain weight. It also contributes to the development of insulin resistance. Excess sugar also triggers free radical production in our bodies and can lead to chronic disease development and tissue and blood vessel damage.

Sugar has about fifty-six other names that it goes by. Glucose, fructose, high fructose corn syrup, maltodextrin, sorbitol, agave, maple syrup, barley malt, malt syrup, dextrose, sucrose, raw sugar, and rice syrup are just a few. It is very important to familiarize yourself with these names, so you can recognize when they are in the foods that you may choose to eat. Hidden sugars exist in a lot of foods that you may not think of as having sugar, or where you may not be aware of the amount.

Just when you thought you were eating healthy, here are some foods that contain hidden sugars that could sabotage your weight loss and/or blood sugar control goals:

Fruit-flavored yogurt	Dried fruits
Granola bars	Soda (Pop) drinks
Salad dressings	Pasta sauces
Nut milks	Peanut butter
Canned fruits in syrup	Barbeque sauces
Frozen meals	Marinades

As a diabetic, it is very important that you monitor your blood glucose level if consuming these foods to determine the effect that they may have on your blood sugar level. Depending on the manufacturer, the amount of added sugar may vary.

The increase in the consumption of processed foods has also led to the obesity epidemic. Yes, they are quick and convenient and easily microwaveable, but have you ever thought of what was taken out and what was put into those foods to increase the shelf life? Many processed starches act as sugar once they are broken down in your body. Processed starches are or are found in things like white flour, white rice, pasta, enriched flour, tapioca, cornstarch, and many breakfast cereals.

Let me emphasize: if you don't already, you need to start reading food labels. In 2010 the Obama administration, thanks to the efforts of the former First Lady Michelle Obama, passed a law calling for a change to the food labeling system. It called for improvements in clarity, accuracy, and consistency of food packaging labels. The new labels put emphasis on the serving size, the amount of servings per container, and the number of calories; the amount of added sugars now has to appear on them as well. This allows you, the consumer, to have the correct information to make healthier food choices.

I'm sure there are a variety of reasons as to how we have allowed ourselves to end up this way. Many people may not have the financial means or access to stores that sell fresh fruits and vegetables or other healthy options. One's culture, environmental factors, genetics, and medical conditions may all play a role in weight gain and obesity. Whatever the reason, it is good that we are becoming aware of the problem now and educating ourselves on the effect that certain foods have on us as a society. Taking action now will hopefully bring about the much-needed change to our bodies, those of our children, and those of the many generations to follow.

INSULIN RESISTANCE

Insulin resistance has also been linked to the weight gain and obesity problems and, as previously mentioned, can eventually lead to prediabetes, type 2 diabetes, strokes, heart attacks, and some cancers. Insulin's normal function is to help glucose get into the cells to be used for energy and the building of muscle. Insulin also promotes the storage of excess sugar as fat for later energy needs. Insulin resistance happens when the cells stop functioning properly and the glucose is unable to get into the cells.

Let's see how this happens. You eat a meal that is refined and highly processed. This meal contains a large amount of carbohydrates, and these carbs are broken down into glucose. The presence of glucose in the bloodstream signals the pancreas to release the insulin. The insulin, as the gatekeeper, signals the insulin receptors on the cells to open and let in the glucose. The glucose is then available to be used for energy and muscle building. When blood glucose remains high, the pancreas releases more and more insulin to try and help get the amount of glucose in your bloodstream into the cells. This process continues as long as there is excess glucose until the receptors stop responding to the insulin's signals. That leaves a lot of glucose in your bloodstream and excess insulin floating around. The excess insulin then signals for the excess glucose to be stored in the liver and fat cells, mainly in the abdominal region, to be used for energy needs later. The development of insulin resistance occurs slowly over the years, with the continuous consumption of carbohydrate-rich meals fueling the reaction. Like hypertension, it can be considered a silent killer, as it is causing damage that you are not aware of until you have developed prediabetes or type 2 diabetes. So, as you have heard before, it is our diet that is the root of the problem. The foods we eat and the choices we make are contributing to the problem of obesity and the development of associated chronic illnesses.

Whatever the reason, we are now aware of the problem; we are now aware of the sheer magnitude of its reach and the effect obesity is having on the health of our nation. It is affecting our friends, our families, our children especially, and perhaps even you individually. It is my intent to give you the knowledge and tools you need to help combat diabetes, weight gain, and obesity, for the health of you, your family members, and ultimately our nation.

CHAPTER 3

Managing Diabetes

Getting the diagnosis of diabetes can trigger a lot of different emotions within you. Hearing my doctor give me the news, saying "Your test results came back and you have diabetes," hit me like a ton of bricks. I was like, "Who, me?" as if someone else was in the room. I instantly felt mad, disappointed, devastated, and sad. I thought to myself, how could this happen? I did all the right things. After my mom passed away because of complications from type 2 diabetes in 2008, I was determined to not get diabetes. I hired a personal trainer and started working out four or five days a week. I got on a healthy meal plan, made some other lifestyle changes, and lost twenty-one pounds. Yes, I went from 178 pounds to 157 pounds. Wow, right? I just knew I was on the right path to being healthy. But five years after that I was diagnosed with gestational diabetes. The diabetes had returned!

The doctor had become the patient. Initially I was in denial, refusing to accept the diagnosis. My doctor wanted to start me on metformin. I said, I'll just try and treat it with more dietary and lifestyle changes. I worked out more, I cut down on the carbs, I drank more water—anything to not take the meds. I was still in denial. It's true, doctors are the worse patients! I would check my fasting blood sugar (FBS) in the morning, but I would get readings of 160 mg/dL, 170 mg/dL, or 175 mg/dL in spite of my efforts. I knew what that meant as a physician, but didn't want to accept it as a patient. My hemoglobin A1c was 7.6 percent, when normal is less than 5.7 percent. I finally realized that I needed to start the meds and get serious about my health. I needed to manage my condition. I needed to learn how to live with diabetes.

What is a hemoglobin A1c? This is the test that your physician will order to monitor how well you are controlling your blood glucose levels. It refers to glycalated hemoglobin. Hemoglobin is the protein part of the red blood cell (RBC) that carries oxygen. When there is glucose in the bloodstream, it binds with the hemoglobin, thus becoming glycalated. The greater the amount of glucose in the bloodstream, the more hemoglobin is glycalated. On average, RBCs live sixty to ninety days. The hemoglobin A1c thus measures the average glucose levels over the previous two to three months. If you continuously have carbohydrate-rich meals, this yields excess glucose in the bloodstream and your hemoglobin A1c will reflect that.

Hemoglobin A1c

Normal = < 5.7%

Prediabetes = 5.7%–6.4%

Diabetes = > 6.5%

I have found that, like me, many of my African American patients are in denial about their diagnosis at first. The emotions that I felt and experienced are shared by many. I realized that a lot of patients know they have the disease, but don't know the right things to do to manage it. They may or may not take their medicine for a variety of reasons. They eat all the wrong foods. They don't check their blood sugar. They don't go to the doctor for regular checkups. That's how they ended up in the emergency department seeing me. Usually they had signs and symptoms of uncontrolled diabetes, including high blood sugar levels. When I would ask why, a lot of them told me they didn't know what to do. Some said they thought they were doing the right things, and some even said they didn't care, that they weren't going to do anything, and that you had to die from something! I realized that perhaps there was a disconnect between the diagnosis, the education about the disease, and the proper lifestyle changes needed to manage diabetes. Many patients stated they were confused and unsure about where to go or who to turn to for help. It is my hope that the information shared with you in this book will serve as a catalyst for you to take control of your health. Learning all that you can about diabetes and its complications will hopefully serve as motivation to start living that healthy diabetic lifestyle.

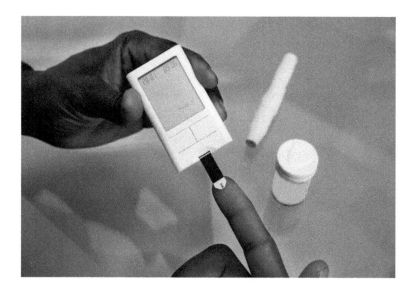

When you have diabetes, it is very important to check your blood glucose level regularly. Your doctor will tell you how often based on the type of diabetes you have and your treatment plan. By checking your blood sugar regularly, you have the information to provide to your doctor so they can put you on the right type of medicine and the proper dose. Blood sugar checks can also let you know how certain foods and activities affect your blood glucose level. Diabetics who take insulin or are on an insulin pump may have to check their blood sugar three or more times a day. If you are an athlete, work out, or lead an active lifestyle, then you need to check your blood sugar level after a period of activity to see what effect it has on your blood glucose. Exercise tends to lower blood glucose; you want to be careful so you don't experience a hypoglycemic (low blood sugar) moment and pass out.

Creating a set schedule to follow may help you remember when to check your blood sugar level. For type 1 diabetes you may need to check your blood sugar before meals and snacks, before and after exercise, and at bedtime. In general, for type 2 diabetes you should check it before meals, after exercise or working out, and at bedtime. Keep in mind, this schedule is not etched in stone and you might need to adjust it based on your individual needs and circumstances; also, remember to consult your doctor before making any changes to your routine. The following is the general normal range for blood glucose levels; however, your physician may give you different target levels that they want you to follow.

Normal Blood Glucose Readings

Non-Diabetics	Diabetics
Fasting: 80–99 mg/dL	Fasting: 80–130 mg/dL
Before meals: 80–99 mg/dL	Before meals: <130 mg/dL
After meals: 80–149 mg/dL	After meals: < 180mg/dL

Keep in mind when checking your blood sugar levels after eating that you have to wait at least 2 hours after the meal. Checking it before waiting that time will give you an elevated level that is not the number that is needed to gauge your treatment plan properly. Again, I want to stress the importance of checking your blood glucose level regularly. It puts the power in your hands as you take control of your health. Being empowered with this information is a big step toward managing your diabetes the right way. You want to make sure that your blood sugar isn't going too high or too low. If it is, then you know that something is wrong, and some changes need to take place or you need to visit your physician.

It is best to keep a log of your readings so you can share the info with your diabetic care team. If you are old school, you can keep the readings in a logbook or notebook; if you are tech savvy, then there are a variety of blood glucose monitoring apps available to use on your cellphone. Why is checking your blood sugar really important? Because by knowing your numbers and keeping them in the appropriate range, it helps to prolong or even prevent the onset of complications associated with diabetes.

CHAPTER 4

Complications of Diabetes

This is one of the most important chapters in this book. It is important because I want you to focus on the long-term complications listed. I want you to share this info with your family and friends. I want you to take heed yourself. The long-term complications listed here are what happens when diabetes goes untreated or is not treated properly. When you have diabetes and your blood glucose remains high, it has a lasting negative effect on your body. It causes damage to blood vessels and nerves that supply your vital organs and limbs. The damage, once it occurs, is unfortunately not reversible.

You might wonder, how specifically does this happen? The elevated blood sugar, over time, causes weakening of the blood vessel walls. The capillaries, which are small blood vessels, begin to leak blood and fluid. As a result of this leaking, the blood vessels are not able to carry the important oxygen and nutrients to the vital organs and nerves. Elevated blood sugar also causes free radicals to develop, and they also cause damage. It is felt that there are multiple factors that lead to the development of these complications. Things like uncontrolled blood pressure, high cholesterol, genetics, and smoking may also play a role.

As previously stated, this damage does not occur overnight. It takes years and years of carbohydrate toxicity for the insulin resistance to develop and become type 2 diabetes. It then takes even more years of poorly controlled diabetes for these complications to occur. This is why it is so important to identify prediabetes early so you can make the necessary changes, like weight loss and healthier eating habits. It is equally important if you are already diagnosed with diabetes that you, too, focus on losing weight, developing healthier eating habits, and monitoring your blood glucose levels. This is the main reason I am writing this book. It is to inform you that diabetes is real, and the ultimate effect it can have on your body is detrimental.

I watched this devastation firsthand with my mother, who was a type 2 diabetic. She had gestational diabetes while she was pregnant with my younger sister. It went away, but then came back in her mid-thirties. She also had hypertension and smoked cigarettes. As a child, I didn't really pay much attention if she took her medicine regularly or not. I do, however, remember as her adult daughter, the doctor, when I asked if she was taking her meds; the answer I got blew me away! I'll get to her answer in a moment. She wore glasses and had gone to the ophthalmologist because she was having trouble with her vision and seeing floaters. The doctor diagnosed her with diabetic retinopathy and referred her for laser surgery. At that time, I was away completing my residency training in Washington, DC. I wasn't there to ask the pertinent questions about the severity of her retinopathy or to get the particulars about the surgery, such as, what were the other options, and what were the risks?

My mom was fifty-seven years old when she went in for laser surgery and came out unable to see the way she had when she went in. Her vision right after surgery was blurry and she could only see the big E on the vision chart; that's the one at the very top of the chart. She was declared legally blind at fifty-seven years old! Her eyesight continued to worsen and she ultimately lost all sight. For a person like my mother, this was life changing, to say the least. My mother had been very active and very independent. She soon became less active and more dependent. Imagine, if you will, what it is like to suddenly lose your eyesight. Close your eyes right now; experience the darkness that your new world becomes. This is the darkness that my mother lived with daily for the next eleven years of her life. The destructive disease process continued and she went on to have both her legs amputated, then she developed kidney failure that required dialysis. Strong as she was, she dealt with these long-term complications of her diabetes for eleven years, but ultimately she succumbed to the complications and passed away in 2008. My mom was sixty-eight years old when she died.

Maybe you or someone in your family, or even someone in your close friend circle, can relate to my mother's story. Perhaps you are the caregiver to someone who is suffering from some of those same complications. Maybe you have heard about the complications and have thought, "It will never happen to me." Well, I certainly hope not, but perhaps my mother thought the same thing. Remember that conversation that I had with her, when I asked her if she had been taking her meds? She told me, "I was, but then I ran out and never had the time to go back to the doctor to get more." Whaaaatt? You can't do that!! What do you mean you didn't have time? I was completely blown away! I wondered how long and how many times she had taken those medication breaks. I wondered if she had been informed of the complications of the disease she was diagnosed with. I wondered if she was told which foods to eat and which to avoid. I wondered if she was told to make some lifestyle changes to improve her quality of life. I wondered, if I was there and more involved in her care before she lost her sight, would it have made a difference? I wonder . . .

My mother's story is my sole motivation for myself as I learn to live with diabetes, and it is my motivation for writing this book for you. Through my practice, I have heard the same answer that she gave and more from my patients. Some take the meds but continue to eat all the wrong foods. Some don't know how or when to take their meds. Some don't take the meds and don't care what happens. Some say, "I'm controlling it with diet." Some continue to smoke. Some go to the doctor regularly and some don't. Many of them never check or monitor their blood sugar levels.

Below are some of the long-term complications of poorly controlled diabetes.

DIABETIC EYE DISEASE

There are three main disorders, collectively referred to as diabetic eye disease, that can affect the eyes of diabetics: cataracts, glaucoma, and diabetic retinopathy. People with diabetes are twice as likely to develop eye disease as people without diabetes. While cataracts and glaucoma are not exclusive to diabetics, they do commonly occur in people with poorly controlled diabetes; diabetic retinopathy is only found in people with diabetes.

In a normal eye, your lens is clear and lets in light to the retina, the light-sensitive tissue in the back of the eye, allowing you to focus and see clearly. When a cataract develops, that lens becomes cloudy and the proper amount of light does not get to the retina, causing your vision to become impaired, making it clouded, blurred, or distorted. Normally, cataracts develop slowly over time, and the risk of development increases as we age. With diabetes, however, this cataract development occurs due to the excess level of glucose in the body, which accumulates in the front part of the eye and forms deposits within the lens. These deposits can soon make your vision appear opaque. Once a cataract develops and affects your vision, preventing you from performing your normal activities of daily living, it has to be surgically repaired. The cloudy lens is removed and a clear, artificial lens is put in its place.

Symptoms of Cataracts

- Poor night vision

- Sensitivity to light

- Seeing halos around lights

- Fading or yellowing of colors

- Patches of blurred vision

- Need for bright light to read

Glaucoma is a disease of the eye that is caused by a buildup of pressure within the eye. This pressure buildup develops when the fluid flow in the eye becomes blocked. Neovascular glaucoma is a rare type of glaucoma that is most commonly associated with diabetes. When new, abnormal blood vessels grow on the iris (the colored part of your eye), they block fluid flow, and the buildup of fluid causes increased eye pressure. As is the case with diabetic retinopathy, which I will discuss below, the growth of new blood vessels is the causative factor, but with neovascular glaucoma they grow on the iris, not the retina. Neovascular glaucoma is difficult to treat, but laser surgery has shown some promise.

Symptoms of Glaucoma

▶ Peripheral (side) vision loss

▶ Headache

▶ Eye pain

▶ Nausea or vomiting

▶ Red eyes

▶ Halos around lights

Diabetic retinopathy is the most common cause of blindness in adults. It is caused by damage to the blood vessels that supply the retina with the necessary oxygen and nutrients. Diabetic retinopathy is separated into two types: non-proliferative, or early, and proliferative, or advanced. In non-proliferative diabetic retinopathy, the damaged blood vessels in the eye begin to swell and leak fluid. In severe cases, this may develop into proliferative diabetic retinopathy. In this advanced form, because the blood vessels are damaged, new blood vessels form to try and compensate. These new blood vessels are fragile and don't allow proper blood flow. This leads to scarring and destruction within the eye.

Non-proliferative (Early)	Proliferative (Advanced)
Damaged blood vessels leak	New blood vessels grow within the retina
Retina or macula begins to swell	New blood vessels are abnormal
	Bleeding vessels cause scarring

Symptoms of Diabetic Retinopathy

▸ No symptoms early in disease

▸ Seeing floaters or dark spots

▸ Difficulty seeing at night

▸ Blurred vision

▸ Loss of vision

▸ Difficulty distinguishing colors

So who is at risk for developing diabetic eye disease? Anyone with diabetes can develop it. At least half will develop some form during their lifetime. The longer you have diabetes, the greater the risk. Unfortunately, the various diabetic eye diseases are now being seen in children and young people, which is earlier than expected and often due to poor diabetes control. Prevention is the key! It is therefore very important to control your blood sugar levels, work to lower your hemoglobin A1c level, and keep your blood pressure within a normal range. Also, you should visit an ophthalmologist annually for checkups. The **ophthalmologist**, who is the specialist for diseases of the eye, will perform a thorough exam and be able to detect any early signs of cataract development, pressure changes, or retinopathy development. When detected early, there are medications that can be used and treatments that can be done to save your vision. But if you don't go, you won't know. Detection and prevention are key to prolonging and/or preventing the onset of blindness. Take control of your health and your destiny. Don't lose the gift of sight that you have been blessed with.

DIABETIC PERIPHERAL NEUROPATHY (DPN)

DPN is a diabetic complication that can develop in the upper and lower extremities. It is the most common complication of diabetes. Continuously elevated blood sugar causes damage to the nerves near the surface of the skin. It generally starts in the legs and feet and then progresses to the hands. It is believed to manifest in the legs and feet first because the nerve fibers there are the longest and most numerous. This damage affects your sensation of touch, temperature, and pressure. This can manifest as either an increase or a decrease in sensation. If you have a decrease in sensation, it means you can't feel cold, heat, or pressure in your legs, feet, or hands. This is why diabetics are at an increased risk of developing diabetic foot ulcers. You get a cut or sore that you don't feel or know is there and it continues to worsen into an infection. The symptoms with DPN are usually worse at night.

Symptoms of Diabetic Peripheral Neuropathy

▶ Burning pain

▶ Stabbing or electric shock sensations

▶ Numbness (loss of feeling)

▶ Tingling

▶ Muscle weakness

The symptoms of diabetic peripheral neuropathy may present themselves differently in each person. It is estimated that approximately 60 percent of people with diabetes will develop some form of DPN. The progression of DPN is slow and happens over years of chronic elevated blood sugar. It also generally starts showing symptoms as diabetics get older. The damage, once it is done, can't be reversed. But all is not lost; you can delay the onset or prevent worsening of the disease by monitoring your blood sugar levels, eating the right foods, and keeping your blood sugar within a normal range. Regular visits to your primary care doctor can also help, because they will do an exam and test for the development of peripheral neuropathy.

DIABETIC NEPHROPATHY

Diabetic nephropathy, also known as diabetic kidney disease, is the number one cause of kidney failure, also known as end stage kidney disease (ESKD). Diabetic kidney disease develops slowly and progressively over the years. It is the chronic loss of kidney function. At least a quarter of people with diabetes develop diabetic nephropathy. African Americans, Hispanic Americans, and American Indians are at increased risk for this development.

Healthy kidneys work to remove waste and toxins from your blood. They also remove excess water from the body as well. The waste and water become urine, which is stored in the bladder until you go to the bathroom and release it. Chronically elevated blood sugar causes damage to the blood vessels and glomeruli (filters) within the kidneys. The damaged kidneys begin to leak protein (proteinuria). As the damage gets worse, sodium, potassium, water, and toxins stay in the body. With complete failure, the body develops swelling, fluid overload in the lungs, and cardiovascular events, ultimately leading to death if not treated.

Your doctor will do a blood test called the serum creatinine; this is used to determine your glomerular filtration rate (GFR). The GFR tells how well your kidneys are functioning. There are five stages of the degree of damage seen with diabetic kidney disease.

DKD	GFR level
Stage 1	> 90
Stage 2	60–89
Stage 3	30–59
Stage 4	15–29
Stage 5	< 15

The onset of symptoms generally starts five to ten years after the disease begins. There is no symptom development early on, but symptoms will begin to manifest as the destruction continues. Often, the first symptom reported is frequent urination at night, or nocturia. As the disease progresses, further symptoms begin to appear.

Symptoms of Diabetic Kidney Disease:

▸ Swelling of the hands, feet, and face

▸ Trouble sleeping or concentrating

▸ Poor appetite

▸ Nausea

▸ Weakness

▸ Extremely dry skin

- Itching (in ESKD)

- Drowsiness (in ESKD)

- Muscle twitching

- Abnormal heart rhythms

The following are risk factors that increase the likelihood of people with diabetes developing kidney disease:

- Uncontrolled high blood pressure

- Poor control of blood sugar

- High cholesterol

- Type 1 diabetes with onset before age twenty

- Past or current history of smoking

- Nerve damage to the bladder

- A family history of diabetic nephropathy

Once end stage kidney disease develops and your kidneys stop functioning to remove toxins and waste, there are several treatment options. If you meet certain qualifications, then you may be placed on the kidney transplant list. If you are fortunate enough to find a matching donor, then the transplant can happen as scheduled and arranged by the transplant team. If not, you will be required to start kidney dialysis until a donor kidney becomes available.

There are two types of dialysis. Peritoneal dialysis occurs inside the body. The waste and water are removed from the blood and cross a semipermeable membrane into a dialysis solution in the abdomen. This process is continuous, and the solution has to be emptied four to five times a day.

Hemodialysis occurs outside of the body. The blood is drawn out of your body and pumped through the dialysis machine. While in the machine, your blood is passed through the dialyzer and dialysis solution. The waste and water are removed and the cleaned blood is returned back into your body. Hemodialysis typically takes four hours and has to be done three times a week for the rest of your life, or until a kidney transplant is done. Hemodialysis is usually carried out at a dialysis center, but treatment at home may also be an option for some people. Once hemodialysis is required, it greatly changes the spontaneity and quality of life that you once led. You now have to add this treatment regimen to your schedule three times a week. It also affects travel, as you will have to make arrangements for dialysis treatment in the city or country you are traveling to if your trip is longer than a weekend.

Although these treatment options exist, early detection and prevention is the key! Visit your doctor for regular checkups. It is equally important to keep your blood sugar and blood pressure under control. If you smoke and you have diabetes, quit now! In the long run you'll appreciate the improved quality of life that you will live.

CHAPTER 5

7-Step Diabetes Management Plan

1. Get Informed

2. Get Support

3. Get Food

4. Get Active

5. Get Trim

6. Get Ready

7. Get Stress Free

This list serves as a guide to help you with making the proper and necessary lifestyle and eating habit changes that will help improve your life by controlling your diabetes.

GET INFORMED!

Since you have this new diagnosis, you want to educate yourself with as much knowledge and information as you can. Meet with a diabetes educator. Research on the internet and find trusted sources to help you gain a better understanding of diabetes and prediabetes. Read books or sign up for informational blogs or podcasts on diabetes. It is very important to ask your physician questions. I feel that some patients are reluctant to ask questions for fear of looking dumb or feeling embarrassed. You know, it was once said to me that "a question is not a dumb question if you don't know the answer!"

Become familiar with the medications you have to take; know what they are and what they do. Knowing the side effects of your medication is also helpful. It is important to learn about hemoglobin A1c, to learn what it means and how it is measured. Once given your A1c number, you should keep it in mind as you work to decrease it. Knowing this number gives you an idea of how well your diabetes is being managed.

GET SUPPORT!

Now that you have a diagnosis of diabetes, it is important to build a support team. This is one of the most important steps you can take toward managing your diabetes. Besides your primary care physician, your support team should consist of:

Diabetes Educator—It is often helpful to find a diabetes educator to assist in giving you the information you need to understand diabetes. They are also a great source for getting the latest up-to-date info.

Dietician—A dietician can teach you about the proper foods to eat that will help you keep your blood sugar levels within a well-controlled range. They may also be able to give you recipe ideas and cooking tips so you can learn how to cook healthy, tastier, diabetic-friendly meals.

Pharmacist—Your pharmacist will assist you with getting your prescribed medication and answer any questions you have about the medication. Staying with the same pharmacist is also helpful because they can monitor for dangerous drug interactions. Your pharmacist can help you to understand your medication regimen. Knowing when and how to take your medication is key to the success of managing your diabetes. Having a good relationship with your pharmacist is valuable, because they are a reliable resource that you can turn to when questions arise about your medication when your doctor is not available.

Podiatrist—A podiatrist is a doctor who specializes in the feet, ankles, and lower legs. They can educate you on diseases and disorders that affect those areas. They will provide preventive care and help you prevent foot and lower limb complications. You should visit your podiatrist at least once a year to be monitored for sores or ulcer development. If you are already dealing with a foot issue, then you may have to see them more frequently. Early detection is the key to preventing diabetic foot ulcers and infection ultimately leading to amputation. Aside from visiting the podiatrist, you should be monitoring your feet as well. If you have developed decreased sensation in your legs and feet, you may not realize that you have a sore or injury. If you are unable to examine your feet, then get a family member to help you. They should be looking for any redness, cuts, cracks, or sores that may have developed. Each year, over 65,000 limbs are amputated due to complications from diabetes. Regular visits to your podiatrist can decrease your risk by 85 percent. As I said before, early detection is key to helping you continue to live a very active, complication-free life.

Ophthalmologist—An ophthalmologist is a medical doctor who treats diseases of the eye. They are not to be confused with an optometrist, who is the eye doctor that treats your vision with corrective lenses. In other words, an optometrist is your prescription eyeglasses doctor. They may detect some changes in your eye and refer you to an ophthalmologist. The ophthalmologist performs a comprehensive eye exam that can detect systemic diseases like high blood pressure, diabetes, stroke, and cancer. Sometimes an ophthalmologist can diagnose diabetes even before a person knows they have it. The ophthalmologist can also perform surgery for various eye diseases if needed. Again, the ophthalmologist is a very important member to have on your team. It is recommended that you visit the ophthalmologist yearly for a checkup. You should definitely see them sooner if you are experiencing problems with your vision, like spots, floaters, or blurry vision. Early detection today is the key to saving your eyesight for tomorrow and many years to come.

Dentist—A dentist is very important because they can detect inflammation and/or infection in your mouth. As a diabetic, you are at an increased risk of developing periodontal disease. Increasing age and poor blood sugar control increases your risk for gum disease. The bacteria that is in your mouth sets up shop in and around your gums. The diabetic body is not able to fight off the bacterial invasion as it normally would, so inflammation and/or infection may develop and persist.

You may notice that your gums bleed when you brush your teeth; this is a sign of gum inflammation. Periodontal disease is the most common dental disease affecting those living with diabetes. If left untreated, periodontal disease can destroy your gums and the bones holding your teeth in place, causing you to lose your teeth. Regular visits to the dentist are important, as your dentist can screen you and detect any problems of gum disease or bone loss. They can also perform professional deep cleanings that help slow the progression of periodontal gum disease.

Chronic infection of the gums leads to an increase in your blood sugar levels. When the body is trying to fight off an infection, it perceives this as stress and releases cortisol and glucagon. These stress hormones cause the liver to release glucose to supply energy, thus constantly keeping blood glucose levels elevated. Research suggests that treating gum disease improves blood sugar control in patients with diabetes. This helps to lower your blood glucose levels and ultimately helps to lower your hemoglobin A1c. Early detection, treatment, and prevention is key to maintaining your healthy smile and controlling your diabetes. It is recommended that you visit the dentist at least every six months for a checkup and cleaning. You might require more frequent visits depending on the degree of periodontal disease that you have. It is also important to floss after each meal and brush your teeth at least two times a day to prevent plaque buildup between visits.

Therapist—Getting a diagnosis of diabetes can be very devastating for some. It unleashes a lot of emotions that you or your loved ones may not know how to deal with. You may experience anger, fear, denial, anxiety, or depression. You might feel resentful about having the disease or about the lifestyle changes that you are going to have to make. You might experience anxiety about the possible diabetic complications that might affect you. Don't worry, as these feelings are normal and natural; however, it might help to talk to someone to put everything into perspective.

Studies show that people with diabetes are 1.5 to 3 times more likely to suffer from depression and/or anxiety. So when should you seek the help of a therapist? If you are newly diagnosed and feeling overwhelmed or have any of the feelings above, then it is a good idea to meet with someone early on. It is best to seek a therapist or psychologist who is experienced in counseling diabetics.

Now, some people may be too proud or ashamed to seek help from a mental health professional. However, it is important to note that your mental health plays a major role in your overall physical health and wellbeing. You might consider finding a mindset coach or enlisting the help of your family and friends as part of your support team. Also consider connecting with other people who have diabetes; you can share your stories, trials, and tribulations with one another. Select someone to be your accountability partner; you can both motivate and keep each other in check while managing your diabetes. If you are religious and know that prayer works, then get yourself a prayer partner or prayer team to help you. Managing your diabetes is a daily struggle that you must learn to live with. Having that special person that you can turn to when you are feeling mentally drained and defeated is an important part of successfully managing your diabetes.

GET FOOD!

As a newly diagnosed diabetic, you will find that you have to look at food differently. You now have to focus your attention on food. You want to become a mindful eater. You want to be aware of the nutritional value and sugar content of what you choose to eat. You want to become aware of how certain foods affect your body and your blood sugar. Quite frankly, food played a big part in how many of us ended up with type 2 diabetes. As I explained earlier, because of the years of carbohydrate toxicity that we exposed our bodies to, we ended up with weight gain and type 2 diabetes increasing at a rapid and steady rate. So, now that we are aware of the problem, it is time to make some corrective changes that will benefit you and your family in the long run.

By making several key changes to the foods that you eat, you can essentially reverse your diabetes. If you are diabetic, then making these changes to your lifestyle and eating habits could delay or prevent the onset of many of the complications associated with uncontrolled diabetes. If you are prediabetic, then changing your eating habits now could prevent you from developing type 2 diabetes later. If you are overweight and on a lot of medicine, you could lose weight and possibly get off all of your meds. Perhaps you have heard a popular quotation about food that states, "Let food be thy medicine and medicine thy food." The wrong food has been the problem, but the right food can be the solution.

It is very important to get as much fiber as you can. Currently, American adults consume about fifteen grams of fiber a day. Total dietary fiber intake should be twenty-five to thirty grams a day from food. Adding thirty grams of fiber to your daily intake can help you lose weight, lower your blood pressure, lower your cholesterol, and improve your body's response to insulin. There are two types of fiber, soluble and insoluble. Soluble fiber dissolves in water and becomes gelatin-like as it passes through your intestines, thus slowing the absorption of sugar and improving blood sugar levels. It also makes you feel full longer, thus causing you to take in less calories. Insoluble fiber stays in its fibrous form and bulks up your stool, helping food pass through your digestive system. This helps you stay regular and wards off constipation. Plant-based whole foods like fruits, dark vegetables, and whole grains are a good source of fiber to add to your diet. Apples, oranges, strawberries, and bananas have around four grams of fiber per cup. Raspberries have eight grams of fiber per cup. Although good for fiber, be mindful of the natural sugar content in a banana: a medium-sized one has ten grams of sugar. For vegetables, the darker the color, the higher the fiber content. A medium-sized artichoke has a whopping ten grams of fiber. On average, we should be consuming five to ten servings of fruits and vegetables a day.

Here is a list of fruits and vegetables with a high fiber content:

Pears	Brussels sprouts
Strawberries	Broccoli
Avocados	Raw carrots

Apples	Beans
Raspberries	Spinach
Bananas	Artichokes

As a diabetic, it is also important to avoid concentrated (simple) sugars, found in foods like cakes, pies, sugary drinks, candy, chocolate milk, granola bars, ice cream, maple syrup, jelly, jams, donuts, and sugar-coated cereals. Other foods, like store-bought marinades, barbeque sauce, salad dressings, and spaghetti sauce, also contain high amounts of sugar. We often prepare our foods or use these things as condiments without realizing that we are adding at least four grams of added sugar per tablespoon. Consuming breads, bagels, white rice, and white pasta will also cause blood sugar spikes. These starchy foods made of refined wheat flour are broken down into glucose inside the body. Consider eating whole wheat or whole grain pastas and breads instead. This is where reading the ingredients is key, because you want to make sure that it contains 100 percent whole-grain flour, not enriched wheat flour.

Here is a list of high-fiber foods that can increase your fiber intake:

Oats (steel cut)	Chia seeds
Brown rice	Flaxseeds
Quinoa	Sweet potatoes

Almonds	Sprouted grain bread
Walnuts	Dark chocolate (no added sugar)
Macadamia nuts	

It is also important to get an adequate amount of protein in your diet. Protein, along with fats and carbohydrates, is a "macronutrient." This means that your body needs large amounts of it. Protein is an important part of every cell in the body. Protein is the building block used to build muscle, bone, cartilage, skin, and blood. Your body uses protein to build and repair tissue. Protein can also help you lose weight. It reduces hunger and boosts your metabolism. Sounds great, right? Just load up on protein and all your problems are solved! Well, not exactly. Many body builders, athletes, and people looking to lose weight load up on protein to try and reach their goals. The high protein/low carb diets are all the rave, but they may not be helpful for everybody. Yes, if you are highly active then you may require more protein, and may even achieve some short-term results. However, it is advised not to continue this eating regimen for more than six months. Such a diet has been shown to be associated with low calcium, potassium, magnesium, vitamins, and antioxidants because you are not getting these vital nutrients from the foods you eat on this restrictive diet. This could lead to heart disease, osteoporosis, stroke, and certain types of cancer. These diets have also been associated with dehydration, constipation, and weight gain, and it puts you at an increased risk of damage to your kidneys if you stay on it for a long time. While there seems to be no adverse effect on healthy individuals with normal, functioning kidneys, you are more likely to worsen your kidney disease if you have kidney problems already and you start consuming a lot of protein.

It is advised that the average man get fifty-six grams of protein per day and the average woman get forty-six grams of protein a day. You can also calculate the amount of protein you need by your body weight. For an average sedentary person, getting 0.36 grams of protein per pound of weight is recommended. If you are trying to lose weight, then 0.7 grams per pound of weight is recommended. If you are trying to gain muscle, then 0.8 grams per pound of weight is recommended. Generally, active men and developing boys require more protein.

Sources of protein include:

Fish	Eggs	Cheese
Chicken (white meat)	Cottage cheese	Artichokes
Beans	Chia seeds	Tempeh
Nuts	Broccoli	Oats
Whole grains	Lean beef	Quinoa
Tofu	Legumes	Turkey

Please consult your physician, nutritionist, or dietician for individualized advice before starting a new eating plan. They can help ensure that you are on a balanced meal plan that will give you the necessary fats, carbohydrates, and protein for your needs.

Now that you are looking to change your eating habits, you want to purge your pantry and refrigerator of those tempting foods that may not be best for you. This may be hard for you if you have a family with kids or other, non-diabetic adults. They may look at you funny when you start to throw away the cakes, cookies, pies, and ice cream, or wonder who drank up all the fruit juice or ate all of the potato chips and pretzels. Change is hard at first, but doing this will benefit both you and your family members. I understand that you may not be able to get the whole house on board at first, so just take baby steps. Start with you, and maybe by example everyone else will fall in line. If you do all of the grocery shopping and prepare all the meals, then the ball is in your court. Children really have no choice; it is up to you to guide them. If your house is like mine, what I cook is what you eat! Or, you don't eat. After I got diagnosed with type 2 diabetes, I decreased the amount of sweets and carbs that I would bring into the house. I didn't deprive them completely, but my kids still called me the Food Police. In any event, they are better for it.

You also will learn to grocery shop differently. Grocery shopping for some is stressful, but it doesn't have to be. First plan your meals for the week, then make a list of the ingredients to shop for. You may have heard people say, "Shop the perimeter of the grocery store." This means to stay in the outer section of the grocery store, where fresh foods like fruits, vegetables, dairy, meat, and fish are usually located. It is best to select a variety of beautifully colored fruits and vegetables, as well as lean cuts of meat, to fill your basket. It is also best to avoid putting a lot of prepackaged, dried, or canned foods from the center aisles in your basket. These foods are usually highly processed and contain various additives and preservatives that may not be the best choice for your dietary goals. Although not located in the perimeter, the frozen food section is also a good place to choose from for fruits and vegetables. These are usually frozen while fresh and are good options.

As a diabetic, changing your eating habits is one of the best things that you can do to manage your diabetes. So make your mind up today to take charge of your health, to take control of your diabetes, and to dedicate yourself to a healthier way of living by changing your eating habits. Doing this will put you on the proper pathway to reversing your diabetes and improving your quality of life.

GET ACTIVE!

As a prediabetic, exercise can help you lose weight, improve insulin resistance if you have it, and actually delay or even prevent the onset of type 2 diabetes. As a diabetic, exercising is a key part of managing your diabetes and your overall wellbeing. Exercise has been shown to help increase insulin sensitivity, helping your body utilize insulin more effectively. When you exercise consistently, along with maintaining a healthy diet, you can lower your blood glucose and improve your hemoglobin A1c. When you lower your hemoglobin A1c, you could possibly require less medicine or be taken off of it altogether, though you should consult with your physician before stopping or adjusting your medication. It is also important to check your blood sugar before and after rigorous exercise. You want to make sure that your blood sugar is not too low or too high. I advise you to keep snacks handy in the event that your blood sugar starts to drop too low during exercise. I also advise that you consult with your physician or healthcare provider before starting an exercise regimen.

There are two types of exercise that are important when it comes to managing your diabetes: aerobic exercise and strength training. Aerobic exercise relieves stress, improves blood circulation, and reduces your risk for heart disease by lowering your blood sugar and blood pressure and by improving your cholesterol levels. You should aim for thirty to sixty minutes of aerobic activity at least four to five times a week. Make sure that you pick an activity or exercise that you enjoy so that you can remain consistent. Here are some examples of various aerobic activities that you can do:

Running/jogging	Swimming or water aerobics
Cycling	Low impact aerobics
Brisk walking	Roller skating or ice skating
Dancing	Basketball
Playing tennis	Hiking

Strength or resistance training also makes your body more sensitive to insulin and can lower your blood sugar. It helps you build and maintain strong muscles and bones, reducing your risk of osteoporosis and bone fractures. It is known that the more muscle you have, the more calories you burn. Your muscles burn calories even while you're at rest. Strength training also helps to prevent muscle loss or wasting that may occur with aging. Strength training should be done at least two times a week in addition to your aerobic exercise. Below are examples of strength training activities that you can do:

- ▶ Free weights or weight machines at the gym
- ▶ Resistance bands training
- ▶ Calisthenics like sit-ups, squats, push-ups, and lunges
- ▶ Lifting objects at home like water bottles or canned goods
- ▶ Total body circuit training
- ▶ Heavy yardwork or gardening

If you haven't exercised in a while or are new to an activity, then I advise you to start off slowly. For aerobic training, start with five to ten minutes and gradually work your way up to thirty minutes, then forty-five, and then sixty minutes. For strength training, start with light weights and work your way up. For the best results and proper technique, you should hire a personal trainer or physical therapist. Again, it is advisable to speak with your physician before starting any workout program.

GET TRIM!

Many people, when they are diagnosed with type 2 diabetes, are overweight, and your doctor or healthcare provider commonly recommends weight loss as part of your treatment plan. It is often because of excess fat that the insulin resistance developed. With prediabetes, weight loss is definitely the treatment that is recommended and will benefit you the most in the long run. Losing weight makes your body less insulin resistant and will make you better able to use insulin. If you have been recently diagnosed with prediabetes or type 2 diabetes and are overweight or obese, you should start your weight loss journey as soon as possible. It has been said that even losing five to ten pounds of weight can benefit you greatly in the long run. It is especially important, if you carry a lot of excess weight in your midsection, to focus on trimming your waistline. Losing weight can be a challenge; however, it is not rocket science—you simply burn more calories than you take in. You have to identify your *why*. Find out what your motivation is for losing weight, what your motivation is for controlling your diabetes, or what your motivation is for getting healthy and staying healthy. Once you've done that, enlist the help of family and friends, an accountability partner, a coworker, or someone else who can help keep you in check as you embark upon your weight loss journey.

Start by working with a registered dietitian or nutritionist who specializes in meal plans for diabetics and can help you set reasonable and realistic goals. Keep in mind that any weight loss is beneficial. As the development of truncal obesity is associated with the development of type 2 diabetes, trimming the waistline is key to reversing your diabetes. Work on adopting a healthy lifestyle that includes regular exercise and eating well-balanced meals. Diabetes is a disease that you have to fight daily, and to do it properly, lifestyle changes have to be your new way of life. Don't rely on fad diets, gimmicks, or tricks to achieve your weight goals; there is no such thing as a quick fix. There are many advantages to losing weight, such as:

▸ Boosting your energy

▸ Lowering your cholesterol

▸ Protecting your heart

▸ Improving blood sugar control

▸ Improving your hemoglobin A1c

▶ Helping you sleep better

▶ Improving your body image

▶ Improving your self-confidence

▶ Reversing your diabetes

Understand that, when you hear "reversing your diabetes," that is because of all the hard work, sacrifice, and discipline that you put in to achieve your weight goals. The positive results are what lead to the decreasing of your blood sugar and hemoglobin A1c levels. However, if you go back to your old ways of eating, then you will sabotage your results, your numbers will increase, and your diabetes will return. So, once you've reached your weight goals, you have to continue on a daily basis to maintain that weight and keep your diabetes in remission.

Here are some added tips to help you achieve your weight goals:

▶ Stay positive

▶ Don't get discouraged

▶ Set realistic goals

▶ Decrease your portion sizes

▶ Follow your meal plan

- Do weekly meal prep

- Avoid unnecessary snacking

- Cook your own meals

- Keep a food journal

- Exercise regularly

- Never give up!

GET READY!

Getting diagnosed with prediabetes or diabetes can be scary, overwhelming, and outright devastating. Learning to live with diabetes is challenging. It can make you feel confused, out of control, depressed, and anxious. These feelings are totally normal. The journey that is ahead of you may seem daunting, but it is definitely doable. Developing a healthy mindset is key to managing your diabetes and your new, healthy way of living. Mindset is defined as a mental attitude, mood, or disposition that predetermines a person's responses to and interpretations of situations. It is how you look at things and then react. Essentially, you control your mindset, and your mindset affects everything in life, not just your health.

Making the decision to change your eating habits and lifestyle is a choice. Everything you do concerning controlling your diabetes and your new way of living is a choice. Having the ability to change your mindset means you have the ability to ultimately change your life. The mind, body, and soul connection must be in sync for ultimate success. You need to train your mindset to focus on healthy living, clean eating, and a nontoxic lifestyle. Again, you are in control! Diabetes is not the doomsday diagnosis you think it is. Yes, there are complications, both short- and long-term, associated with diabetes, but making the necessary changes now could prevent you from ever experiencing them. Yes, you now have to take medication. Yes, you have to refill your medication when you run out. Yes, there are certain foods that are now off-limits. Yes, you have to meet with a dietitian and follow a meal plan. Yes, you now have to cut out some of your old habits. Yes, you now have to exercise regularly. Yes, you now have to monitor and record your blood sugar. Yes, you now have to prick your finger several times a day. Yes, you now have to go to your doctor's appointments regularly. Yes, you have to lose weight. Yes, and yes, and yes. It seems like a lot, doesn't it? Do not be discouraged or dismayed. I felt the same way at first, but then I made my mind up to learn how to live with diabetes. I decided to learn how to control diabetes and not let diabetes control me. The following are seven steps that I use to develop a healthy diabetic mindset:

1. **Love who you are.** This step is probably one of the most important ones, because it all starts with you. We all struggle at some point in time with low self-esteem or self-confidence. Today's society makes it even harder, as

we look around and compare ourselves to the "perfect image" that is portrayed on television, on billboards, and in magazines. Accepting and loving yourself for the uniquely beautiful person that you are goes a long way toward boosting your self-confidence. You are about to develop life-changing habits that will yield a better version of you.

2. **Believe in yourself.** As you get started on this health journey, you have to believe that you will achieve success with the goals set up before you. It may help to start the day off with positive affirmations. Daily affirmations will help you start your day focused on thinking positive. Perhaps you have heard the saying, "whatever the mind can conceive and believe, it can achieve." In my opinion, no truer words have been spoken. Believe it.

3. **Focus on the positives.** Often in life it is very easy to fall into a negative way of thinking and living. For a healthy mindset, it is essential to focus on the positives. Instead of focusing on what you can't have or can't do with your new lifestyle changes, focus your attention on what you can do. Identify those things or people in your life that you have to be thankful for. Yes, you have diabetes, but be grateful that the lifestyle and dietary changes you make will positively impact your outcome. Negative thinking is a surefire way to sabotage your journey, and quite possibly your results.

4. **Be intentional.** Living with diabetes requires you to be intentional. It is a lifelong journey that requires you to be purposeful. It means that you make thoughtful choices and decisions in your life. It is best to be proactive instead of reactive. To be intentional, you have to map out your goals and devise a plan on how to accomplish them. Practice intentional living every day by asking yourself, and then realizing, why you make the choices that you do. Intentional living every day is about doing the things that are important to you, even when they may not be easy to do. Being intentional makes you feel in control of your life.

5. **Learn from your mistakes.** Making mistakes is a part of everyday life. No one is immune to making mistakes; we are all human. A mistake is usually a wrong action that you can learn from and then correct. The key is to own your mistake and not make excuses. Analyze your mistake and then put into place a corrective action plan. Try not to be so hard on yourself. Making new lifestyle and eating habit changes takes time.

6. **Never stop learning.** Living with diabetes is a lifetime commitment. You should want to gain as much understanding about the disease as you can. There is so much information available to you to assist you while on this journey. There is so much to learn about food, about exercise, about medication side effects, about mindset

development, etc. Never stop being the student; always remain open and willing to learn new information. You can always refer to Dr. Google (or other internet sources), books in the library, pamphlets from the doctor's office, YouTube, or even apps on your phone to discover information that you need or want.

7. **Celebrate your success!** It is important, at the end of the day, that you celebrate your success. No matter how big or small, success deserves to be recognized. Celebrating your success helps keep you motivated and feeling good. It allows you to focus on what you've accomplished and to not dwell on the task ahead. Celebrating success also helps you develop a success mindset. Sharing and celebrating your success with others allows them to recognize your hard work and efforts and may serve to motivate someone else. Celebration helps build your confidence, keep you on task, and fuel you with energy for continued success. So celebrate!!!

GET STRESS FREE!

You want to, when at all possible, minimize the stressors in your life. I know it is easier said than done; however, this is very important because stress plays a role in the weight gain that we experience. When we are stressed, our bodies perceive that we are preparing for battle and go into a fight or flight mode. The stress hormone cortisol is released during this time, causing stored sugar and fat to be released into the bloodstream to be used for energy. The presence of glucose in the bloodstream causes the release of insulin, which makes your blood sugar drop; this causes the brain to signal for the release of more cortisol, setting the stage for a vicious cycle of weight gain. An increase in cortisol also causes you to crave sugary treats and fatty foods. The presence of excess insulin causes the glucose to be stored as fat, further contributing to weight gain, and the cycle continues. Eating certain foods and skipping meals, as we often do when we are stressed, contributes to this cycle. Foods like cakes, pies, ice cream, sodas, high glycemic starches, and even alcoholic beverages can raise your cortisol and insulin levels. These foods, which are high in sugar, trigger the pancreas to release an excess of insulin. The stress that most of us experience nowadays is psychological. It is our perception of and reaction to the various things that affect our daily lives that triggers this stress. As we chronically stay in a stressed state, our bodies will continue to release cortisol. So now you can see why minimizing your stress is an important step in managing your diabetes. To minimize stress, you might try these things:

Remove the stressors. I realize that it may be difficult or impossible to remove certain things that stress you out, like your job, your family, or your financial situation. You may just have to step back and take a vacation from the situation. Going to a local hotel for a brief staycation may also help. You can also work on the way you react to the stressor.

Meditate. The practice of meditation is meant to train your mind to focus and redirect your thoughts. Meditation and mindfulness have been shown to effectively reduce stress and anxiety. Meditation has other benefits as well. It has been shown to improve your sense of wellbeing, improve your cardiovascular health, and strengthen your immune system. Studies have shown that meditation actually decreases the stress hormone cortisol.

Do yoga. The practice of yoga brings together mind and body. It involves breathing exercises, meditation, and various controlled poses designed to bring about relaxation and reduce stress. Yoga has also been shown to reduce cortisol. Other benefits include reducing anxiety and depression and improving quality of life.

Exercise. Exercise is known to increase your overall health and your sense of wellbeing. Physical activity helps to increase the production of the feel-good hormones called endorphins. Exercise improves your mood and causes you to focus and forget about the troubles of the day. Don't have time, you say? Well, make time, for there is no room for stress on this health journey. Consider doing it in ten minute increments for something like interval training.

Write in a journal. When you are stressed, writing down your experiences and reactions can help you better learn how to deal with them. It can give you insight on why you feel or react the way you do when stressed. Writing down your healthy eating and exercise goals might also be helpful, as it will make you more conscious of your intent to live a healthier lifestyle and stay committed.

Listen to relaxing music. Listening to music for a lot of us is second nature. We have been doing it for as long as we can remember. I remember growing up listening to The Temptations, Al Green, Stevie Wonder, Natalie Cole, and so many other great musical artists that my mom would play. When we hear certain songs, they may evoke feel-good emotions or memories. With the advent of cellphones and headphones, now more than ever we see people treating themselves with music therapy. Here's why it works: our bodies have a psychological response to music. Music taps into our emotions, allowing us to feel a certain way. Music has been shown to improve our attention skills. Music enhances learning. And overall, music is motivating, relaxing, noninvasive, and safe.

Get more sleep. In this crazy busy, fast-paced world in which we live, with so much piled on our plates, many of us are sleep deprived. Research shows that not getting enough sleep increases your risk of high blood pressure, heart disease, weight gain and obesity, and diabetes. Sleep deprivation makes you moody, irritable, fatigued, forgetful, and even unable to concentrate. It is recommended that adults get seven to nine hours of sleep per night. Some may need more, while some may be able to function on less; however, you should aim to get at least the shortest recommended amount of seven hours per night.

————— C H A P T E R 6 —————

Herbs and Supplements for Diabetes

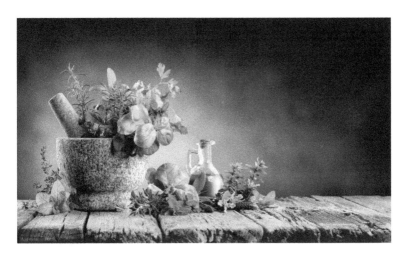

You might have seen a lot of information out there about different herbs and supplements that may help people with prediabetes or type 2 diabetes lower their blood glucose levels.

Research has been done on some herbs and supplements, and they have been shown to have promise in these limited studies. Because of the limited amount of studies, more research needs to be done before herbal supplements can be declared as effective treatments for type 2 diabetes. I just wanted to share with you this information to enhance your knowledge concerning herbal supplements.

Please do not stop taking any diabetes medication you have been prescribed until you are instructed to do so by your physician. Also, some herbal supplements may interfere with your diabetes medication by treating the reverse symptoms, thus making your blood glucose levels worse. **This is for informational purposes only and should not be deemed as an alternative treatment option without first consulting with your physician.**

Aloe Vera—The aloe vera plant has been used for thousands of years because of its healing properties. Studies suggest that the juice from the aloe vera plant can help lower blood sugar in people with type 2 diabetes.

Fenugreek—This herb has been used in the Middle East for thousands of years as a medicine and as a spice. The benefits of this herb have been demonstrated in both animal and human studies, where it was found to have a significant effect on controlling blood sugar.

Curcumin Extract—Curcumin is a bright yellow compound produced by the spice turmeric. Curcumin has been shown to have several benefits for prediabetes and type 2 diabetes. It has been shown to inhibit the free radicals that cause damage to the cells. It has also been shown to help reduce the risk of developing diabetes symptoms and complications. Curcumin also reduces high blood sugar, hemoglobin A1c, and insulin resistance.

Green Tea Leaf Extract—Green tea has been shown to be a safe and effective antioxidant. A study done in Japan showed that green tea reduced the risk for the onset of type 2 diabetes. In type 2 diabetics, green tea improved glucose tolerance and decreased blood sugar production. Green tea has also been shown to have a positive effect on the blood vessels by reducing any overgrowth of these vessels that may occur. This is thought to have a significant effect on preventing diabetic retinopathy. Green tea is also known to promote fat breakdown and boost metabolism.

Ginseng—The herb ginseng has been used as a traditional medicine for more than two thousand years. Studies suggest that both American and Korean red ginseng may help to lower blood sugar levels in people with diabetes. In one study, the extract from the ginseng berry was able to improve insulin sensitivity and normalize blood sugar in mice.

Cinnamon—There have been a number of studies on cinnamon. They have shown that cinnamon can slow stomach emptying and lower postprandial (after a meal) glucose levels. It also has been shown to reduce glucose levels in type 2 diabetics who have poor diabetic control on medication. Cinnamon may also be helpful in lowering insulin levels, hemoglobin A1c, blood pressure, and free radical formation. There are two specific types of cinnamon that have been shown to have the best effect on diabetes symptoms. These are Cinnamonium cassia (Chinese cinnamon), the most common commercial type, and Cinnamonium burmanii (Indonesian cinnamon). I know, I just got a little scientific on you.

Chromium—Chromium has been shown to bind to and activate the insulin receptors on cells in the body, which improves insulin resistance. Chromium supplements have been shown to lower blood sugar levels, lipids, hemoglobin A1c, and insulin in diabetic patients. It is also said to decrease your appetite for sweets. Be aware, though, that high doses of chromium may worsen insulin sensitivity in healthy people who are not obese or diabetic.

Magnesium—Magnesium is important for glucose balance and the release of insulin from the beta cells. It also increases the affinity and number of insulin receptors on the surface of cells in the body. It is common for some diabetic patients to be deficient in magnesium. This is because magnesium is excreted out in the urine as a result of high blood sugar levels. When magnesium levels are low, it causes insulin resistance. Studies have shown that when type 2 diabetic patients with low magnesium were given the supplement daily for sixteen weeks, it reduced insulin resistance, fasting glucose, and hemoglobin A1c levels.

Vitamin D3—Vitamin D3 plays an important role in the secretion of insulin and in preventing insulin resistance. Vitamin D3 decreases your blood sugar by increasing the way your body responds to insulin. Studies have shown that people newly diagnosed with type 2 diabetes tended to have lower vitamin D levels than people without the disease. It is believed that an adequate intake of vitamin D3 may prevent or delay the onset of diabetes and decrease complications for those who already have diabetes. As Americans, we may not always get adequate amounts of vitamin D, also known as the sunshine vitamin. Our lifestyles and eating habits play a big role in this deficiency. We work long hours indoors, we stay covered up with clothing, and, when outdoors and exposed to the sun, we slather on sunscreen. Now, I'm not saying to quit your job, walk around in your birthday suit, and stop using sunscreen; I'm just pointing out that the sun is a good source of vitamin D.

Using supplements may assist you in maintaining your blood sugar goals. As I stated before, it is important to consult with your physician before adding these supplements to your treatment regimen. If given the okay, some of these supplements can definitely serve as an adjunct in assisting to keep your blood glucose in the desired range. You might consider seeing a naturopathic physician who can help you utilize herbs and supplements properly. Naturopathic medicine is a system that uses natural remedies to help the body heal. It uses many therapies, including natural herbs and supplements, massage, acupuncture, exercise, and nutritional counseling. The ultimate goal, however, is to change and enhance your diet so that you are ultimately receiving the vital nutrients and vitamins that your body needs. I personally use a lot of fresh herbs when I prepare my meals. I even grow my own herbs in my indoor herb garden. Fresh herbs are great because they help to enhance the flavor profile of your food as well as give you some added nutrients.

CHAPTER 7

Making Time for the Diabetic Lifestyle

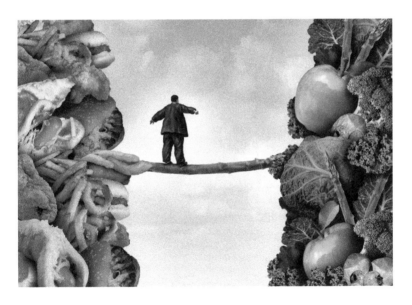

If you've recently been diagnosed with prediabetes or type 2 diabetes, you're probably thinking, oh my God, not another thing that I have to worry about. If you're the caretaker of a friend or a loved one, you too probably feel like you are facing an insurmountable task. In today's fast-paced, scurry-about, always-something-to-do world, your schedule is probably already full, with no room for anything else. You might say to yourself, I don't have time in my day for another thing, and you might be right. Getting a diagnosis of prediabetes or diabetes and making the decision to change your eating habits and live a healthier life is a choice. It is a choice that you make, hopefully with the intent to stick to it to improve your quality of life in the long run. It's all about choices and decisions. I used to tell my kids when they were growing up that choices and decisions dictate the outcome of your life and what you have to live with. When you make a decision, it is your choice to carry it out, and carrying it out means being able to live with the consequences of your decision.

I hear people say, "I'm too busy and I don't have time for that." They say, "My job keeps me busy, my kids keep me busy, my friends and coworkers keep me busy." They say, "I don't have time to cook," "I don't have time to grocery shop," "I don't have time to exercise," "No, I didn't check my blood sugar," or "I forgot to take my medication." During my many years of working in the emergency department, these are some of the statements that my patients made to me. When I heard them say these things, I would ask them, "Well, now do you have time?" "Do you now have time to deal with this complication of diabetes that has developed because you didn't take the time before?" I asked the men, who are most times the worst when it comes to taking care of themselves, "Do you have time now that you are blind and can no longer go to work, to that job that had you too busy?" Or I would say, "Do you have time now that your kidneys have failed and you need to be placed on dialysis for three days a week?" I know that may sound harsh, but that is the passion that I treated my patients with. I would tell them straight up what could happen, just in case no one else has. As a physician, it frustrates me to no end that people don't take their health seriously until it's too late. Preventive care is so much better than reactive care.

My mother, bless her heart, didn't stop smoking and start taking her medications until she lost her eyesight. The day she lost her eyesight, she stopped smoking cold turkey. And mind you, she had smoked for thirty years and had tried several times to quit, but to no avail. I just wish that I could stand on the rooftop and shout, "DIABETES IS A SERIOUS DISEASE, PEOPLE, AND IT CAUSES HARM TO YOUR BODY EVERY DAY IF YOU DON'T TREAT IT PROPERLY!" People would probably look at me like I was some crazy lunatic, but at least I would have their attention for that moment. Some people would get the idea and listen further, but others would go about their day and tell their family members when they got home about the crazy lady on the roof, and that would be the end of it.

All jokes aside, learning to live with diabetes is a serious matter. I tell my patients that time is of the essence, and that you make time for those things that are important to you. I let them know that I am a wife, a mother, and a physician who is a type 2 diabetic. I share with them the fact that I have a husband, four very active and involved kids, and a dog, and although I am a busy emergency medicine physician, I make time. Though it may not always be easy or even convenient, I make time to go grocery shopping; I make time to make my family home-cooked meals that they enjoy, because I want them to be healthy, too. I make time to make the right food choices when faced with temptation. I make time to check my blood sugar and take my medicine every day. I make time to exercise at least four to five times a week on a good week. I make time because I am as important to my family as I am to myself, and I want to make sure that I am doing my part to positively affect my quality of life for years to come.

A lot of people say to me, "Girl, I don't know how you do it; it seems like too much to handle." Sometimes I feel the same way, but what I know to be true is that God does not put more on you than you can handle, and I live by that, day by day. All it takes is having a plan in place to help guide you along. What works for one person may not work for another. In a previous chapter I gave you the seven steps that I feel will help you manage your diabetes. You may have to tweak certain things so that it works for you, your situation, and your lifestyle. However, if you commit to making changes for yourself or your loved ones, you will certainly be well on your way to controlling diabetes.

I talked about food earlier, and how what we choose to eat as a diabetic plays a major role in managing our blood glucose levels and weight goals. Healthy meals don't have to be bland or boring, and you shouldn't feel like you have to keep eating the same thing. You just have to be adventurous and willing to try new foods. If you don't normally cook at home, you should start. By cooking your own meals, you know exactly what ingredients were used and you control the amount of salt, sugar, and fat in your dish. I will usually plan meals for the week ahead, writing down the meals I plan to cook for dinner and what I will take for lunch. I also consider what snacks I want for the week, too. I then make a shopping list and set about my task. I actually enjoy grocery shopping; I really like the super gourmet-type stores that have every spice or ingredient you need to make any ethnic dish you desire. I actually enjoy cooking very much. I come from a family of good cooks. I like taking a recipe and reconfiguring it to make my own, healthy, tasty interpretation of it. I used to prepare a big meal at the beginning of the week, thinking that it would free me up with one less thing to do for a couple of evenings; however, my husband and kids would eat the leftovers for lunch or an after-school meal and then be looking at me to cook something else for dinner! Ha! So, clearly, you have to adjust your plan and program to fit your family dynamics, all while keeping it doable for you.

Cooking and eating with diabetes is a lifestyle, not a diet or a short-term quick fix. Once you really get into it, you will find that it is really not that bad. You will automatically start choosing the right foods and cooking meals that will help you achieve your goals. When getting started with your eating plan, you can consider using the Plate Method, which is recommended by nutritionists. This is simply where you fill half the plate with non-starchy vegetables, a quarter of the plate with a protein, and the other quarter of the plate with whole grain and fiber-rich foods. You can also add a small piece of fruit on the side. Each of your meals should contain these components; make sure that you stay mindful of your portion sizes.

Don't look at it as if it is a chore; look at it as a way to enhance your life or that of your loved ones for the best. Change is always hard at first, so don't try and do everything all at once. It takes around twenty-one days of doing something before it becomes a habit. So, start today and see where you are in two months; measure your progress, and don't forget to celebrate each milestone along the way!

Consider using these smart food swaps as a way to get started on your healthy eating journey. Good luck!

SMART FOOD SWAPS

Swap Out White Rice for Brown Rice

Whole grain brown rice has more nutritional benefits than white rice. Brown rice has twice as much fiber, zinc, and selenium, as well as increased amounts of folate potassium, vitamin B3, and magnesium.

Swap Out Red Meat for Fish

Red meat is known to be high in saturated fats and calories. Fish is lower in fat than red meat and is a rich source of healthy omega–3 fatty acids, which have been found to improve heart health. It is also loaded with important nutrients like protein, vitamin D, iron, zinc, magnesium, and potassium.

Swap Out Butter and Margarine for Olive Oil or Avocado Oil

Cooking with butter or margarine exposes you to high levels of saturated, unhealthy fats. They also contain sodium and solid fats. Olive oil or avocado oil are both good sources of monounsaturated fats.

Swap Out French Fries for Baked Sweet Potato Fries

If on a weight loss journey, you should really stay away from fried foods. French fries from white potatoes will definitely spike your blood sugar. Sweet potatoes, however, have a lower glycemic index than white potatoes.

Swap Out Salt for Herbs

You can use fresh or dried herbs and spices to help improve the taste of your food. Try and experiment with fresh herbs like basil, thyme, parsley, cilantro, dill, etc. The list is endless, so go ahead, be creative and be surprised at what you make.

Swap Out White Pasta for Spaghetti Squash

Spaghetti squash is a great low-carb alternative to pasta. It has two grams of fiber and only forty-two calories per one cup serving. It is also a good source of calcium, potassium, magnesium, and niacin.

Swap Out Creamy Salad Dressing for Balsamic Vinaigrette

Certain salad dressings are rich in saturated fat, added sugar, and calories. It is very important when choosing a store-bought salad dressing that you read the label and choose one that supports your dietary goals.

10 FOODS TO HELP CONTROL DIABETES AND AID WEIGHT MANAGEMENT

1. **Fatty fish**—Fish are a great source of omega–3 fatty acids, which are great for improving heart health, decreasing inflammatory markers, and reducing triglycerides. It's also a great source of high-quality protein to help you feel full. Salmon, mackerel, herring, sardines, and anchovies are some examples. Aim to eat at least two servings per week.

2. **Eggs**—A great source of protein, eggs are a great food for keeping you full. Eggs have been shown to decrease inflammation, improve insulin sensitivity, and increase the good cholesterol HDL. This means eating the whole egg, including the yolk, as the benefits that you get from eggs are due to the nutrients found in the yolk. Eggs have been

shown to reduce the risk of heart disease and promote good blood sugar control.

3. **Turmeric**—This is a spice with powerful health benefits. Its active ingredient is curcumin, which has been shown to reduce blood sugar levels and inflammation while also protecting against heart and kidney disease.

4. **Leafy Green Vegetables**—Spinach, kale, and other leafy vegetables are very nutritious and low in calories. They are a good source of vitamin C and other minerals, as well as antioxidants. One study showed that increasing vitamin C intake reduced inflammatory markers and fasting blood sugar levels in patients with type 2 diabetes.

5. **Greek Yogurt**—This yogurt has been shown to improve blood sugar control and reduce the risk of heart disease because of the probiotics it contains. It also may contribute to weight loss because of its high protein content that decreases your appetite and calorie intake. Remember to eat the plain version, with no added fruit or sugar.

6. **Apple Cider Vinegar**—Apple cider vinegar is reported to have a vast number of health benefits. It's been shown to improve insulin sensitivity and lower fasting blood sugar levels. It may also reduce your blood sugar response by as much as 20 percent when consumed with high carbohydrate-containing meals. It is also believed to slow stomach emptying, which will keep you feeling

fuller longer. If you decide to start using apple cider vinegar, start with one tablespoon mixed in a glass of water
per day, then gradually increase to a maximum of two
tablespoons mixed in water per day.

7. **Chia Seeds**—Chia seeds have been shown to reduce
    blood pressure and inflammatory markers. They are high
    in fiber but low in digestible carbs, so they won't raise
    your blood sugar. The fiber works to lower your blood
    sugar levels by slowing down your stomach emptying
    and affecting the rate at which food is absorbed in your
    G.I. tract. The fibrous seeds also keep you feeling full lon-
    ger and reduce hunger. Chia seeds are rich in omega–3
    fatty acids. They are also a good source of protein, calci-
    um, and various other healthy minerals. They are a great
    addition to your morning smoothie, as well as to other
    foods and recipes.

8. **Flaxseeds**—Flaxseeds are an insoluble fiber made up of
    lignans, which have been shown to decrease the risk of
    heart disease and improve blood sugar control by de-
    creasing hemoglobin A1c. These seeds also improve in-
    sulin sensitivity. The high fiber seeds keep you feeling full.
    They, too, are a great addition to your morning smoothie.
    Be sure to refrigerate your seeds after opening them.

9. **Nuts**—Studies have shown that the regular consumption
    of nuts may reduce inflammation and lower blood sugar,
    hemoglobin A1c, and LDL (bad cholesterol) levels. All

types of nuts contain fiber and are low in digestible carbs, there are just some that have more than others. The ones with the lower amount of digestible carbs per one ounce serving are almonds, hazelnuts, walnuts, macadamia nuts, and pecans. Always be mindful to watch your portions when consuming nuts.

10. **Garlic**—Garlic is one of my favorite herbs. It is delicious, adds so much flavor to your meals, and has health benefits. Several studies have shown that garlic can reduce inflammation, blood sugar, and LDL cholesterol in people with type 2 diabetes. Garlic has also been shown to be effective at reducing blood pressure.

This list is by no means comprehensive, but it should give you a good place to start implementing some of these foods into your eating regimen. Again, these are merely suggestions, and it is advised not to start using these foods without first checking with your physician and/or your dietitian, as some of these foods and supplements may have an adverse reaction with some of your medication.

The benefits of healthy eating will positively affect your life for years to come. The primary goal of your healthy diet is to supply your body with the vitamins, nutrients, and energy it needs to function, all while maintaining a normal blood glucose level. A healthy, well-balanced diet will help you achieve and maintain your desired weight, improve or control your cholesterol, and avoid the complications associated with diabetes and weight gain. As you embark upon this health journey, you will be training yourself to enjoy a new variety of foods that are tasty and good for you. Consider food to be the building blocks and you the architect, building a healthy new you one meal at a time.

———— CHAPTER 8 ————

Living Your Best Life!

I'm sure that you have heard the phrase "Living your best life." You have probably read it somewhere or seen it on the internet, maybe even heard it in a song. You might even use it yourself, as it has become a pretty popular phrase lately. But what does it really mean? The definition for you might be quite different than for the next person. It might even be quite different from mine.

Of course, your definition is based on your interpretation of "living" and "the best life." Some would say that having the ability to wake up every morning is living. Some would say having a big house or driving a fancy car is living. Others might say having a nice job and being able to support their family is living. Some might also say that being in love is living. These same interpretations can be applied to the meaning of "the best life" as well. However, to go further, the best life for some could mean getting your college degree, getting married and having a family, taking a trip around the world, etc. Again, it's a personal interpretation that is individually applicable. In my opinion, it's about identifying your *why, what,* or *who*; it's about living in your purpose; and it's about being optimistic about the outcome and making choices that lead toward that desired outcome. It is when the desired outcome is reached that one might then say, "I'm living my best life!"

In this book I have given you the *what.* You have learned about the various types of diabetes, the cause of diabetes, and the complications that can arise from poorly treated diabetes. I have shared with you my 7 Steps to manage your diabetes, and discussed food as a problem and as a solution. So now you have to identify *your* why, and your why might be different from the next person's. When it comes to making the decision to take control of your life and your diabetes, ask yourself, why are you doing it? Maybe your why is to prevent complications from developing. Maybe your why is to get off all of your medication. Maybe your why is to lose weight and gain more self-confidence. Whatever you why is, let it be your purpose for doing what you do to fulfill it every day. And then there is your *who*; who are you doing it all for? Your who might be a spouse, a child or children, a parent or parents, or even a significant other. Your who, quite frankly, could be you, because after all, it starts with you and it ultimately affects you.

Let's look at being optimistic about the outcome. Optimism goes a long way toward a positive and successful outcome. As I said before, your mindset has a direct effect on the results. Starting each day with a positive attitude will help you push through, even when times are tough. Believing in yourself and staying focused helps you keep your eyes on the prize. Staying motivated helps you make the proper choices that will ultimately yield you the prize. When temptation arises, reflect back on your *why, what,* or *who* to gain that inner strength that keeps pushing you forward. The ultimate prize is the desired outcome. What is your desired outcome concerning diabetes? Do you want to change your lifestyle and eating habits? Do you want to not have to take insulin shots? Do you want to start an exercise program or increase your activity? Do you want to decrease your risk of heart disease, stroke, or kidney failure? Do you want to prevent prediabetes from becoming type 2 diabetes? Whatever your desired outcome is, it can be achieved when you commit yourself to doing all that you can to combat the problem, put into action the solution, and go on to live your best life!

Living with diabetes is a lifetime commitment. It is easy for us to slack off once our goal is met, but with diabetes we can't let our guard down. We have to stay the course and fight the fight! Until there is a cure, we have to continue to educate the masses. We have to continue to equip people with the information that allows them to make the proper decisions concerning their health. Until there is a cure, we have to continue to let people know that making healthy changes to your lifestyle and eating habits can reverse type 2 diabetes. We have to let people know that, if you are put on medication to treat your diabetes, you must take it as prescribed by your doctor until they take you off of it. People need to know that going to their primary care physician regularly is a must. So, until there is a cure, I will continue to stand on the rooftop of the tallest building and shout, "DIABETES IS A SERIOUS DISEASE, PEOPLE, AND IT CAUSES HARM TO YOUR BODY EVERY DAY IF YOU DON'T TREAT IT PROPERLY!"

Thank You!

Thank you for taking the time to read this book. I sincerely appreciate each and every one of you. I hope that you have gained a better understanding about the disease diabetes, its complications, and how to prevent them. Please continue to spread the word; make diabetes the topic of conversation at the coffee shop, the dinner table, or even as you stand in line at your favorite store. Knowledge is power, so share this book and the information in it with anyone you know that may benefit from it. As a physician, I feel that it is so important to continue to educate the masses, both in the exam room and beyond. Diabetes is a serious disease and people need to know that. Hopefully, you now feel empowered with the knowledge of how to live with diabetes successfully. God bless you and may you be well.

Dr. Sharita

To stay up to date with me and all the helpful information I have to share, please follow me on the social media sites below:

www.facebook.com/DrSharitaMD

www.twitter.com/DrSharitaMD

www.linkedin.com/DrSharitaMD

www.instagram.com/DrSharitaMD

www.pintrest.com/DrSharitaMD

www.google.com/+DrSharitaMD

www.youtube.com/user/DrSharitaMD

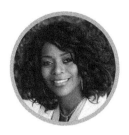

About the Author

Dr. Sharita E. Warfield (Dr. Sharita) is a highly respected, board-certified emergency medicine physician, as well as a nationally recognized author, speaker, clinical instructor, and weight management consultant. She obtained her bachelor's degree from Central State University, a master's degree from Tennessee State University, and her medical doctorate from Wayne State University School of Medicine.

Dr. Sharita completed her internship and residency training in emergency medicine at Howard University. She is originally from Detroit, Michigan, and now resides in Houston, Texas, with her husband, Dr. Brett Warfield, and their four children. She is the founder and CEO of Warfield Medical Group, PLLC, which works to raise awareness about chronic diseases, especially diabetes, obesity, and weight management. In her spare time, Dr. Sharita enjoys cooking, baking, and creating recipes. Aside from cooking, she also loves to spend time cycling, going on nature walks, shopping, and traveling.

To learn more, visit her website at DrSharitaMD.com

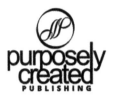

CREATING DISTINCTIVE BOOKS
WITH INTENTIONAL RESULTS

We're a collaborative group of creative masterminds
with a mission to produce high-quality books to position
you for monumental success in the marketplace.

Our professional team of writers, editors, designers,
and marketing strategists work closely together to ensure
that every detail of your book is a clear representation
of the message in your writing.

Want to know more?
Write to us at info@publishyourgift.com
or call (888) 949-6228

Discover great books, exclusive offers, and more at
www.PublishYourGift.com

Connect with us on social media

@publishyourgift